Caregiver CHOICES

An empowerment guide to help you navigate the journey together

Caring Ambassadors Program

Contributing Authors

Ann Broderick, MD, MS and Fred LaBrecque

Editors

Cindy Langhorne-Hatfield and Fred LaBrecque

ISBN: 978-0-578-53370-4

Caregiver
CHOICES

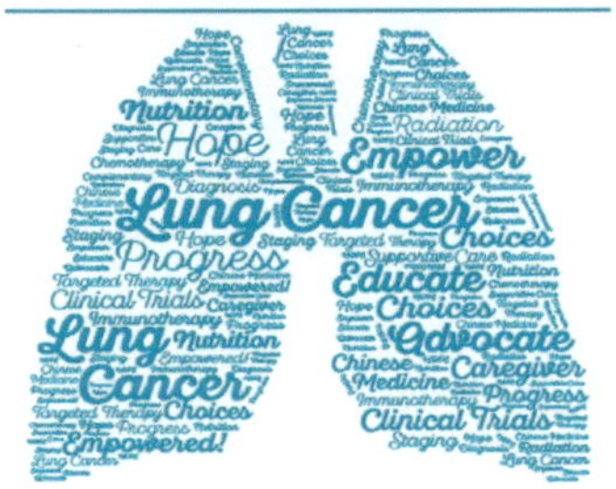

CONTENTS

	Introduction	i
1	Who is a Caregiver?	1
2	Understanding Your Feelings	3
3	Getting Help	9
4	Taking Care of Your Loved One	11
5	Planning Ahead	21
6	Understanding Lung Cancer	25
7	Treatments for Lung Cancer	31
8	Lung Cancer Health Care Team	35
9	Questions for the Health Care Team	43
10	Prognosis	45
11	Key Decision Points in Care	47
	Conclusion	49
	Caregiver Resources (online)	51
	Afterword	55
	About the Contributing Authors	57
	About the Editors	59
	Acknowledgements	61

Caregiver
CHOICES

INTRODUCTION

Right now, someone you care about has lung cancer. This is a tough time.

Caregiver Choices is a resource for all those who find themselves in the role of caregiver for someone who has been diagnosed with lung cancer. We hope that this book will help you support your loved one with lung cancer and take care of yourself throughout your future together.

A life-changing illness brings much more than the symptoms of a disease. Challenges and potential opportunities arise, as well. New perspectives, values, and inspiration can emerge if they are welcomed and fostered. For example, unexpected illness and a stroke of inspiration gave rise to the Caring Ambassadors Program.

In 1993, Ken Giddes was diagnosed with lung cancer. After an extensive period of treatment, Ken's cancer appeared to be in remission. As Ken reflected on his experience, he pondered how to use his experience to benefit others. With a strong belief in the power of people helping people, Ken and his employer, Jim Possehl of Republic Financial Corporation (RFC), came up with the idea of a program to help people struggling with life-changing illnesses get the support, help, and information they needed. In 1997, Ken and his employer turned their inspiration into reality. The Caring Ambassadors Program was founded at the same time as its first disease-specific program, the

Caring Ambassadors Lung Cancer Program.

Ken spent the last years of his life working as a Lung Cancer Caring Ambassador, giving talks about his experiences and being empathetic and encouraging to others who were facing it. Later, his cancer returned, and Ken passed away in January 2001. However, the work he believed in and passionately dedicated himself to goes on.

One of the most meaningful results of Ken's inspiration was the creation of *Lung Cancer Choices*, a patient-focused book that provides information about lung cancer to help people make decisions about their treatment for lung cancer. We are proud of *Lung Cancer Choices* and hope that both you and the person you're caring for will find it helpful.

This book, *Caregiver Choices*, is a companion to *Lung Cancer Choices.* It focuses on you, the caregiver, and all you might face during your experiences. We hope this will not only help you be the best caregiver you can be, but that it will also help you take care of yourself during this journey.

A note on person-first language: you will notice throughout this document that we consistently use the phrase "person with cancer" or other similar terms and that we try to avoid phrases such as "cancer patient" and the like. The difference may seem trivial to you, but listing the person before the disease, rather than the other way around, can be a powerful mental comfort to a lot of people. Nobody wants their lives to be defined by a single thing, especially something like cancer. People who hear themselves referred to over and over as a "cancer patient" may start to feel like cancer has taken over their lives and that it is the only thing that anyone cares about anymore. We do not believe that is true; people with cancer have many other attributes that should be celebrated. By putting the person before the disease, we are telling people with cancer that they are more than their cancer.

Caregiver
CHOICES

CHAPTER 1

WHO IS A CAREGIVER?

If you picked up this book and have read this far, you're probably a caregiver.

Right now, someone you care about has lung cancer. This may be a close or distant relative, a friend, a neighbor, or someone else in your social circle. Regardless of the exact nature of your relationship, if you are taking a supportive role in helping someone with lung cancer, then you are a caregiver.

> *Anyone who helps another person through a tough time is a caregiver.*

The diagnosis of a serious condition such as lung cancer can be stressful, frightening, and overwhelming. Such news often causes the person with the disease to shut down or to freeze in place. In such cases, the role of caregivers is essential. While it may not be your place to make decisions that will impact another's health, you can do everything possible to help the person you are caring for make their own choices. You can help organize and prioritize the decisions that need to be made. You can help provide the best information. You can take over smaller tasks that can get in the way of bigger decisions. You can motivate and inspire. You can help your loved one get moving again or just be there to listen and respond.

Living with lung cancer is not easy, nor is acting as a caregiver for someone who has lung cancer—caregivers can become overwhelmed, too. We hope that this guide, *Caregiver Choices*, will help you navigate the road ahead.

Caregiver
CHOICES

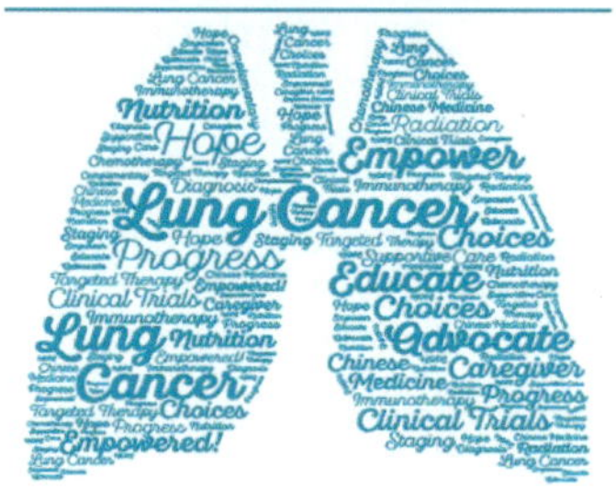

CHAPTER 2

UNDERSTANDING YOUR FEELINGS

Before reading more about lung cancer and the road ahead, stop for a second, and assess how YOU are going to take good care of yourself and manage your own well-being. Think about the emotions that you are experiencing and do not dismiss them. If you fail to take care of your own emotional well-being, you will not be able to be the best possible caregiver.

We are all unique and react emotionally in different ways to stressful experiences. As a caregiver for someone with lung cancer, you may end up having many of the same feelings as the person with cancer. You and your loved one and other caregivers may also respond very differently. Regardless, it is essential that you recognize your own reaction and the reactions of others as valid.

Accept your own feelings and take care of yourself first.

As a caretaker, you may be inclined to act strong for those around you, especially for the person with lung cancer. But being strong does not mean repressing or dismissing your own emotions—it means noticing and caring for your own feelings so that you can be emotionally available to the person you're caring for.

Grief

Grief comes with a loss of any kind. When someone is diagnosed with a serious illness such as lung cancer, patients and their families and friends find their lives turned upside down.

Everyone involved in the life of someone with cancer, including you as a caregiver, will grieve the loss of their routine and their former lives. This grief can emerge even when a cure or years of remission are possible. Often patients and families do not recognize their sadness or irritability as grief, or they grieve privately, not wishing to upset others.

Recognizing grief is part of good self-care. We encourage you to acknowledge your own grief and to share it with those around you. It is likely others are feeling the same emotions and will appreciate the opportunity to share their own feelings.

Grief can show itself in many ways: anger, rejection, sadness, mood swings, irritability, denial—these are just a few of the ways that different people express their grief. Be aware of these feelings in yourself and in others and do your best to channel these emotions in positive and productive ways.

> ***People with cancer often feel grief, and grief can show up in many different ways.***

An excellent place to start when trying to help someone deal with grief is to remember what has helped you and your loved ones get through tough times in the past. Unless you have led an unusually charmed life, it is likely that you have grieved before. Call upon those experiences for ideas. Perhaps when a loved one died, the person you are caring for found an activity that helped him or her through tough times. Maybe he or she enjoyed spending time with family, or dove deeper into religious activities, or just went to the movies with friends. Whatever helped in the past might just help again, even if the cause of the grief was far different from dealing with lung cancer.

Many people who are dealing with grief find that it helps to "get it out". How you choose to take those feelings into the world is entirely up to you. One of the simplest ways is by talking to someone else about what you are going through. As a caregiver, you might be the first one that the person you are caring for turns to. In other cases, it may be more appropriate, comfortable, or helpful to talk with a trained counselor or therapist. Look for a professional who is educated and has experience in helping people deal with grief. Or you could write in a journal. Putting pen to paper can bring relief from grief, even if you never share these private thoughts with anyone else. Finally, one of the simplest ways is to choose an object to focus on that can draw your attention and take the place of your grief. For example, you and your loved one can light a candle of hope together.

While it is important that you help the person you are caring for manage grief, you must also remember that to be the best caregiver you can be, you must also deal with your own grief. You may be surprised to find that the person with cancer wants to hear about the grief that you are feeling and help you through it. Though it may not be the case for everyone, many people who are dealing with a serious illness and managing grief of their own find relief and even joy in helping others. This can be good for both of you. If talking about it seems to help, then speak with each other.

Getting grief "out in front" of you in these ways can help manage it. It is healthy at times to help the other person think about things other than their illness and grief. A simple, discreet way that you can make this happen is by purposely creating casual situations to surround the person with cancer with friends and family. You can gather loved ones in traditional ways that will remind everyone of happy times—lingering over a shared meal is an enjoyable way to create this situation. At other times, putting together a big meal is not necessary and may feel too formal or just be too much work. In that case, hosting a simple movie night with friends and family for a few hours can really help all involved deal with their grief by merely being together. Any reason to gather people who love the person with cancer, and where disease and illness and grief are not the focus, can help raise everyone's spirits.

Finally, it is vital to understand how grief can affect younger people and the ways grief shows up in them. While this is not something unique to lung cancer, it is common for children, or even grandchildren, to be caregivers. Lung cancer is diagnosed mostly in older adults, so children and grandchildren often end up caring for a parent or grandparent. You or one of your caregivers may find yourself in this position, a reversal of roles that can be strange, even shocking. Such situations present their own set of potential problems and call for a frank discussion. Simply noting the newness and oddness of the changing situation can help everyone get past the discomfort. Being honest with each other about your feelings and concerns will help both you and the person with cancer adapt to and even enjoy changes in your relationship.

> ***Join a Caregiver Support Group***
>
> **There are lots of ways to help people feeling grief – finding a positive support group is often a good start.**
>
> **In a support group for caregivers, people may talk about their feelings and trade advice. Others may just want to listen. It may help you to know that you are not alone, and it will give you ideas on how to cope.**

Frustration

Frustration is an emotion that may crop up repeatedly after a lung cancer diagnosis. The person you are caring for may feel frustrated that there are not better treatments to stop or cure the disease. They may be frustrated about the considerable disruptions to daily life that are common for most patients with lung cancer. So many frustrations, big and small, new and old, will appear daily. As a caregiver, you can help avoid or prepare for some of them. For the many trying situations that cannot be predicted, you can help the person with cancer accept the feelings of frustration and move past them.

You will also have your own sort of daily frustrations in your new role as a caregiver, and it is equally important that you recognize and manage your own emotional responses. You will, at times, become impatient, even aggravated, with the person with cancer and, though you may feel tempted to do so, it will not do anyone any good for you to ignore these feelings and allow them to fester. It is a difficult but important challenge to find a productive way to manage the uncertain or even negative feelings that you will have toward the person with cancer. At such times, having your own support system in place is essential. You need to be able to talk openly about your own frustrations, whether to a friend or a professional counselor, so that you avoid bottling up these emotions and maybe damaging your caregiver relationship.

> ***Both the person with cancer and his or her caregivers may feel frustration, resentment, or guilt at times — don't ignore these feelings or let them get in the way of your health.***

Resentment

Another emotional response that may come up again and again with a lung cancer diagnosis is resentment. It is natural and understandable for someone who is diagnosed with a serious disease to resent others. Even if friends and family rally around the person with cancer, the patient may choose to focus on who did not show up to help or who are not doing as much as others. Likewise, as a devoted caregiver, you may want to spend your energy resenting the relatives and friends who are not, in your opinion, doing all that they can to help. As a caregiver, you may resent the person with cancer since you may have given up activities or work that provided needed self-care or income for you. Again, such emotional responses are undoubtedly valid and may very well have some basis, so it is crucial that you admit them to yourself and help the person with cancer to do the same.

You and the person with cancer can help each other move beyond resentments by expressing gratitude to all those who have devoted themselves to providing care. Sincerely and regularly thanking the professionals, family members, and friends who are all acting as caregivers in one way, or another can be a positive practice for all involved.

Guilt

Guilt and blame often come along with the lung cancer diagnosis, in both the patient and caregivers. In our society, there is stigma associated with lung cancer. There are significant exposures that can cause lung cancer (tobacco, radon, and Agent Orange) and not all of them were under control of the person with cancer. Despite any past actions, no one deserves lung cancer, but it is quite possible that the person with cancer might feel this way. This type of guilt can be quite harmful: people who think they deserve to have lung cancer might very well feel that they do not deserve treatment for it. As a caregiver, you can keep an eye out for any signs of such guilt and help the person with cancer get beyond such feeling and move forward with their medical care. Letting the patient share such feelings is a simple yet valuable service that you can provide. It is likely that you and the person with cancer have been spending more time together since the diagnosis—these special moments together can be a real gift. Maybe you have had the opportunity to try out some new recipes when preparing meals for them—it can be enjoyable to experiment in the kitchen. Or perhaps you have become closer to the other people helping provide care—new or closer friendships often come from tough situations, such as caring for someone who is ill. No doubt you will have to work through some trying times as a caregiver, but there are also upbeat parts of the caregiver experience, too. By focusing on the positives, you can help both the person with cancer and you move past the feelings of guilt often associated with a diagnosis of lung cancer.

Caregiver
CHOICES

CHAPTER 3

GETTING HELP

A strong and positive relationship between you as a caregiver and the person with lung cancer can grow in many ways. The beginning is often one of the most challenging parts. Reaching out and asking someone for help can be hard for many people diagnosed with lung cancer, even when they are quite sick and know they could use some support. Now that you have started this caregiver relationship, you both may be tempted to keep your support circle small, to avoid more of the uncomfortable "starter" conversations. Yet, if possible, making efforts to expand your community of caregivers can be so valuable for you and the person with cancer.

As we note in this guide, people with lung cancer need many different types of care, and they appreciate many kinds of support throughout their journey. Even if you have unlimited time, resources, and energy, it is unlikely that you are the best or only person to provide each kind of care and each sort of support at the moment it is required. People with lung cancer find themselves in a world that has been turned entirely upside down. One of the key difficulties is simply finding their way through this new, unfamiliar, and unwelcome world. As a caregiver, one of the first things that you can do is help that person decide what kind of help they need and who might be able to provide it.

> ***If possible, you should not try to care for someone all on your own.***

Making a basic list of ways in which others can give support and matching the right people with the right sort of assistance will let you reach out to them and will help you respond when others contact you. You and the person you are caring for may find that people around you appear with true but vague offers to help. You may frequently hear others say something like, "if there is anything I can do, please let me know." Such offers are heartfelt, and we encourage you to accept them all! If you have thought this out beforehand (remember that list?), it will let you consider the offers and talk about them in a way that is comfortable for everyone involved. Such planning will allow you to accept these offers graciously and in a way that gets things done.

If possible, you should do your best to avoid a situation in which you are the only person giving all the various types of support to the person with cancer. Just expanding your community of caregivers is likely to benefit the person with lung cancer more than any other single thing you do. If the person with cancer resists asking others for help, you should certainly respect their feelings. However, it is best if you can convince him or her that bringing others into the fold is in everyone's best interest.

Help the person you are caring for put together a large group of caregivers who are onboard and have different strengths and the shared goal of helping their friend or family member or coworker or acquaintance or neighbor through the lung cancer journey. Bringing this community together will help the person coping with lung cancer and give much needed support to you as a caregiver.

Caregiver
CHOICES

CHAPTER 4

TAKING CARE OF YOUR LOVED ONE

Patients with lung cancer have a variety of symptoms, and every patient is different. Some common symptoms of lung cancer may be present throughout the course of the disease, some may come and go, and some might not show up at all. As a caregiver, it helps to know about these various symptoms or side effects that may affect their quality of life. The care that is provided with the intent of helping patients cope with these symptoms or side effects is called palliative care, supportive care, or symptom management. Chapter 8: Supportive Care in *Lung Cancer Choices, 5th Edition*, the companion book to *Caregiver Choices*, has detailed information about palliative care for lung cancer patients. Here is an overview from the perspective of a caregiver that we hope you will find useful as you fulfill your role.

Nutrition

- Do not be surprised or upset if the sense of taste of the person with cancer changes from day to day and even from hour to hour. There may be days when he or she does not want a favorite food or says it tastes bad now.

- It is a good idea to keep food within easy reach at all times. That way, the person with cancer can have a snack when he or she is ready to eat. Depending on the preferences of the person with cancer, you could leave a snack-pack of applesauce (along with a spoon) or a favorite protein drink on the bedside table.

- A good rule of thumb when choosing between different foods is to focus on good sources of protein. A lung cancer patient should try to eat at least one gram of protein for every kilo (2.2 pounds) of body weight every day.
- You will probably want to keep urging the person with cancer to eat more than he or she feels like eating. It is best to offer this encouragement as gentle support. That way, it seems much more helpful than pushing them to eat. When there is no appetite, you can suggest that he or she drink plenty of clear liquids.
- The person you are caring for may struggle to eat a lot of food at a time. A good option is to suggest smaller meals more often throughout the day.
- It is important to talk openly and frankly about ways to manage "eating problems". Having regular conversations can help both of you feel more in control and can avoid any major issue

Exercise

Many treatment regimens for patients with lung cancer have side effects. In general, a physically fit body can better tolerate drugs and treatments. So, you can encourage the person you are caring for to think about getting more exercise. Many studies have shown that physical activity and exercise can improve fatigue, quality of life, cardiorespiratory fitness, pulmonary function, muscle mass and strength, improve sleep quality, and decrease anxiety and depression in people living with lung cancer.

A 2018 systematic review of studies found preoperative exercise was effective in reducing postoperative complications and length of hospital stay in patients with lung cancer. Cardiorespiratory endurance and muscular strength have been shown to be independent predictors of survival.

Anything that has the potential to improve health outcomes is worth exploring. The American Cancer Society and American College of Sport Medicine recommend avoiding inactivity and suggest people living with cancer should engage in regular physical activity. Consider talking about exercise with the person with cancer and encouraging him or her to speak with a medical professional about appropriate activities. You may consider adding a kinesiologist, physical therapist, or cancer exercise specialist, and an oncology dietician to your team. There are often barriers to exercise for people living with lung cancer. It is important to make a flexible program that is aligned with their needs and preferences. Start easy and make sure they are listening to their body.

Exercise can help us feel better about ourselves just by making us feel more energetic.

All aspects of health are connected. Exercise can improve your physical health and mental health. Helping the person with cancer develop an exercise plan and sticking with it can become one of your key roles as a caregiver. Better yet, join in, it might also help you manage the physical and mental stress of being a caregiver.

Pain

Pain is a warning sign that something is not right. If muscles, bones, or organs are damaged, then the pain is usually a constant ache, throbbing, or tenderness in one spot. This type of pain responds to medicines that treat the source of the symptoms.

Nerve pain is quite different and requires different medications. Patients often describe the pain as shooting, burning, electric, and intense. Unlike muscle pain, nerve pain can come out of nowhere—the person with cancer may not have any pain one moment and seconds later be in unbearable pain. Opioid medications (those containing or based on morphine) usually do not help.

It is important for the person with cancer to keep a pain diary. This simple journal is a place for the person with lung cancer to describe his or her pain to the medical providers honestly. It is an excellent way to get them information as they manage the pain of the person with cancer. As a caregiver, you can offer to help write the pain journal, making it as easy as possible for the person with lung cancer. It does not have to be complicated. A notebook that lists times, basic descriptions of pain, and how the person responds to pain medicines will do the trick.

Be vocal and honest about your pain.

Pain diary: Take this to your appointments.
https://www.cancer.org/content/dam/cancer-org/cancer-control/en/worksheets/pain-diary.pdf

Opioid Medication and Addiction

Medicines called 'opioids' come from morphine (made from a type of poppy), or they are artificial forms made to have the effects of morphine. When used for a long time, a patient will become used to the effects of the drug. Medical providers skilled in the use of the opioids will monitor their use carefully, switch opioids when necessary, and taper the patient off them when they are no longer required. When the medications are taken for pain, addiction is unlikely.

However, as a caregiver, it is vital for you to know that certain patients are at high risk for opioid addiction. For example, patients who have a drinking problem or are cigarette smokers or who have a family history of alcoholism are at a higher risk for opioid addiction. Likewise, people who have mental health issues are more likely to develop an addiction to opioids. In all likelihood, people with lung cancer with these increased risk factors will still be prescribed opioids, but they should be monitored for safety more closely. As a caregiver, you can help make sure that the person you are caring for is monitored appropriately so that he or she does not become addicted.

It is also critical that we all keep the communities safe. Keep the opioids out of reach and locked away from young children, teenagers, and visitors to the home. Do not store them in the medicine cabinet in the bathroom. Unfortunately, people with cancers are often targets for people with addiction.

Constipation

If the person you are caring for will be taking any opioid pain medication, it is essential for them to take a laxative at the same time to counteract the constipating effects. Products containing senna and bisacodyl are common, but there are others, too. Polyethylene glycol, sold under the brand name Miralax, is another one. Others, including docusate and Colace, are not usually effective, so encourage the person with cancer to explore other options.

Laxatives are not necessary if the person with cancer has a feeding tube delivering their nutrition.

Managing constipation can seem embarrassing for many lung cancer patients to discuss. Depending on your relationship, he or she may be hesitant to talk about it. However, ignoring this issue can lead to emergency room visits.

Shortness of breath

Many people with lung cancer have shortness of breath, whether or not they have had surgery as part of their treatment. Be alert for any sudden shortness of breath they have and report it to their health care team as soon as possible. Sudden shortness of breath may be a sign of something else that needs treatment right away, such as a blood clot or fluid in the lining around the lungs. You can make sure that the person with lung cancer is aware that sudden shortness of breath might be a significant change and that they need to take it seriously.

If the person with cancer was a smoker or exposed to secondhand smoke, he or she may have chronic obstructive pulmonary disease (COPD). In such cases, patients with lung cancer often need to use an inhaler to reduce the inflammation and narrowing of the airways in their lungs.

If the shortness of breath is not changing much over time, there are some effective therapies to manage the symptoms:

- Pulmonary rehabilitation is an exercise designed to strengthen breathing muscles and other muscles. It can be very effective, though many people with lung cancer find it hard to tolerate.
- Low dose opioids can help reduce the disturbing feeling of not being able to catch a breath. When used for this, drugs are given at very low doses compared to treating pain.
- One simple method for relieving shortness of breath is a fan. Direct the air toward the person's face if that is comfortable. There are receptors on the human face that sense air movement and send signals to the brain to reduce the sensation of 'air hunger'.
- Some people with lung cancer will need to use oxygen to manage their shortness of breath. Suggest that the person with cancer talk over this option with the health care team. If oxygen is required, encourage the person with cancer to use the oxygen. If oxygen saturation measurements remain below 88% for prolonged periods, other complications can result.

Nausea

As a caregiver, it can help to understand the basics of when the person you are caring for may become nauseated (have an upset stomach). There are four main causes of nausea in patients with lung cancer:

> ***Take medications with small amounts of food.***

- Many drugs, including pain medicines, especially those used in chemotherapy, can cause nausea.
- Many patients with lung cancer experience some stomach or upper intestinal irritation, which can cause them to feel nauseated.
- The mind of a person with lung cancer can influence the body to feel nauseous. Anxiety about upcoming chemotherapy treatments, called

anticipatory nausea, commonly occurs in lung cancer patients. Also, the brain can sometimes perceive pain as nausea.

- Some lung cancer patients will feel vertigo or motion sickness, which can lead to feelings of nausea.

Each type of nausea is treated differently. You can help the person with cancer recognize the cause and provide his or her health care team with the information they need to give effective treatment.

Fatigue/Weakness/Loss of Appetite

To one degree or another, everyone with lung cancer feels fatigue (tiredness). You can help the person with cancer deal with fatigue in several ways. Encouraging the person with cancer to keep moving and helping with sleep are basic things that can reduce fatigue. Preventing weight loss and making sure they know it is good to ask for help are also worthwhile.

Even if the person with cancer takes all these steps, fatigue may still become an issue caused by a variety of things. The body creates cytokines in response to inflammation, and these cytokines cause fatigue, weight loss, and loss of appetite. Cancer that is increasing in size needs nutrients for its rapidly growing cells and can "steal" energy from the rest of the body.

When helping figure out how best to handle fatigue, there are some basic questions that you can bring up for discussion with his or her support team and health care providers:

- Sleep problems: is the patient's sleep disturbed because of pain, shortness of breath, treatment side effects, or anxiety?
- Mood: is the person with cancer worried, depressed, or blue?
- Treatment: is the person with cancer more fatigued after radiation or chemotherapy? Are there any medications causing the person with cancer to feel more tired?
- Could anemia be causing the fatigue?

- What type of exercise can the person with cancer safely do?
- Is the person with cancer a candidate for pulmonary rehabilitation?
- Could low oxygen in the blood be the problem?

Role of Palliative Care

A palliative consultation can be beneficial for patients with advanced lung cancer. Especially if diagnosed with late-stage disease, you should encourage him or her to seek out a palliative care consultation. There is evidence that patients who receive a palliative care consultation within eight weeks of diagnosis have a higher quality of life, report fewer depressive symptoms, and live slightly longer. This study was a surprise to many in the medical community, who had thought that palliative care was the step leading quickly to hospice.

> ***For more information on palliative care visit GetPalliativeCare.org***

At its best, palliative care eases symptoms and helps patients with lung cancer choose their personal treatment goals at crucial decision points. These decisions are made with their entire health care team—surgeons, radiation oncologists, and medical (chemotherapy) oncologists. As a caregiver, you may find a palliative care consultation especially helpful in defining your role and making sure that you are doing everything possible to support the person with cancer. At first, the person with cancer may not want to explore palliative care, but they can ask for a palliative care referral at any time.

Encourage the person with cancer to investigate palliative care when he or she feels ready. See *Lung Cancer Choices, 5th Edition,* Chapter 8: Supportive Care

Integrative Medicine

Integrative medicine is a total approach to care that involves the patient's mind, body, and spirit. If the person with cancer is at all open to pursuing various health care approaches, we suggest that you encourage him or her to explore how integrative medicine can be used to treat lung cancer. Integrative medicine combines conventional western medicine with complementary and alternative medicine (CAM) practices that have shown the most promise. CAM is an umbrella term used to describe a group of diverse medical and healthcare systems, practices, and products that are not generally considered to be part of western medicine. CAM therapies can often help improve the quality of life for individuals living with diseases such as lung cancer and have even been shown to improve health outcomes.

Integrative oncology is a patient-centered, evidence-informed field of cancer care that utilizes mind and body practices, natural products, and/or lifestyle modifications from different traditions alongside conventional cancer treatments. Integrative oncology aims to optimize health, quality of life, and clinical outcomes across the cancer care continuum and to empower people to prevent cancer and become active participants before, during, and beyond cancer treatment.

The person with cancer may be interested in exploring the different healthcare systems from around the world. As you help him or her search for qualified practitioners of CAM therapies, do your homework, just as you should with any health care provider. Encourage the person with cancer to ask questions about the provider's experiences treating people with lung cancer and to ask about what resulted from the methods.

There are many different CAM therapies that the person with cancer might pursue as part of an integrative medical approach to lung cancer treatment. For example, some cancer patients learn to use relaxation techniques to reduce stress during chemotherapy. Others find that acupuncture helps relieve nausea. Many people with various ailments have found that yoga helps them manage pain. Regardless of the CAM therapies that the person with cancer explores, it is important to keep the primary health care team, including all western medical practitioners (the doctors, nurses, and social workers) in the loop. Openness and communication among everyone involved in the care of someone with lung cancer are critical. You can help see that everyone on the health care team stays on the same page. See: *Lung Cancer Choices, 5th Edition*, Chapter 11: Integrative Medicine, Complementary Therapies, and Chinese Medicine in Lung Cancer

CHAPTER 5

PLANNING AHEAD

Finances

A serious medical condition such as lung cancer can create real financial difficulties for both the person with the disease and his or her caregivers. After a diagnosis of lung cancer, the person with cancer may have to take time off work as, to a lesser extent, will caregivers. If you or any of the other caregivers are immediate family members, this situation can create an even tough financial situation for the family. As a caregiver and an advocate, it is crucial to ask questions that will best help the person with cancer to recognize and plan for the fiscal impact of the disease.

The financial issues associated with serious health issues, and with cancer in particular, are not a new problem. Nor are these issues specific to lung cancer. The American Cancer Society has put together an excellent resource regarding the financial impact of cancer, including a list of important questions for the person you are caring for. This resource is available on the American Cancer Society's website: https://www.cancer.org/treatment/finding-and-paying-for-treatment.html

The financial issues that come up with a lung cancer diagnosis do not only concern the person with cancer; these issues can also become important for you as a caregiver. If the person with cancer is a family member, you should consider requesting Family Medical Leave Act (FMLA) paperwork from your employer. The FMLA allows an employee time away from work to assist a family member with medical issues. Make sure that you understand all of the details of your employer's policy; FMLA mandates that employees be given time off of work to care for family members but does not require that it be paid.

It is also a good idea for both you and the person with cancer to talk to any professionals who might help you navigate potential financial difficulties: your banker, your financial advisor, and a social worker. If the person with cancer is a Veteran, it is important to explore what Veteran benefits might be available to support them with the county Veteran Services Officer (VSO). These meetings will help ensure that you understand how you might meet some of these unexpected financial needs through use of retirement benefits, governmental programs, or other means. Having these conversations soon after diagnosis, instead of waiting until you are in the middle of a monetary crisis, can bring peace of mind to the person with cancer and his or her caregivers, including yourself.

Following a lung cancer diagnosis, one of the first things you should do financially is help the person with cancer to closely review any insurance policies he or she might have, to understand what is covered. Pay special attention to deductibles, co-pays, and the out-of- pocket maximum outlined in the policy. Unless you both have a lot of experience or background with complex insurance documents, you may want to request that the insurance provider connect you with a case manager who can explain benefits and address any outstanding concerns.

A lung cancer diagnosis can have a really devastating fiscal impact on younger patients. The younger a cancer patient is, the more likely he or she is to experience financial hardship due to outstanding loans, lack of savings, and insurance status. If you are a caregiver for a younger patient, you may want to help the person with cancer explore any family resources that might be made available to help cover the costs of treatment. Asking for help can be hard but could result in loans or gifts to help with some of the expenses. Often, families and friends will want to hold fundraising events, too, which can increase the circle of care while easing financial strain.

Another useful resource for financial advice is the health care team of the person with cancer. There are probably not financial experts, but these oncologist, nurses, social workers, and other providers have more frontline experience than anyone in helping patients with lung cancer manage all aspects of their care. They may be especially valuable in sharing insider knowledge about assistance programs offered by the American Cancer Society, pharmaceutical companies, and state and federal agencies. Encourage the person with cancer to ask these experienced professionals if he or she might be eligible to receive any financial assistance.

Finally, a simple way to cut down on costs is to help the person with cancer find the most convenient locations for regular tests, treatments, and office visits. If you can work with the patient's health care team to schedule visits in locations that are close to home without sacrificing quality, you will not only combat fatigue and stress, you will save time and money.

Ultimately, your main role as a caregiver regarding financial issues is to make sure that the person with cancer does not ignore his or her financial well-being. He or she may wish to push any money trouble to the side, understandably believing that there are more important things to think about. However, such a mindset can cause small financial issues to grow into big, even major, financial problems. Help the person with cancer get out in front of these money worries and look for assistance when needed. By doing so, you will both stand a much better chance of weathering the financial storm that often comes with a lung cancer diagnosis.

Notes

Caregiver
CHOICES

CHAPTER 6

UNDERSTANDING LUNG CANCER

Lung cancer is a complex disease. Unless you have previous experience with the disease, it is likely that you knew little about lung cancer when the one you are caring for was first diagnosed. It is also quite possible that what you have heard about the disease is inaccurate or misinformed. As a caregiver for someone who has lung cancer, you may find it helpful to have a basic understanding of the disease. The following pages provide a simple overview of lung cancer. Then, if you want to learn more about lung cancer, there are many excellent resources available, including *Lung Cancer Choices, 5th Edition*, at https://LungCancerCAP.org.

Another excellent resource is the National Cancer Institute's (NCI) website, https://cancer.gov; much of the following is adapted from the free resources provided by NCI.

Your Lungs

We will begin at the most basic level. Your lungs are a pair of large organs in your chest that help your body get the oxygen that it requires. Air enters your body through your nose or mouth before it passes through your windpipe (trachea), through each bronchus, and into your lungs.

When you breathe in, your lungs expand with air; this is how your body gets oxygen. When you breathe out, air goes out of your lungs; this is how your body gets rid of carbon dioxide.

The right lung has three parts, called lobes. The left lung is smaller and has two lobes. Inside the chest are two thin layers of tissue called the pleura. One layer of pleura covers the lungs and the other layer lines the inside of your chest; it is as if your lungs are inside two balloons.

Cancer Cells

Cancer begins in cells, the building blocks that make up all tissues and organs of the body, including the lungs. Healthy cells in the lungs and other parts of the body grow and divide to form new cells as they are needed. When healthy cells grow old or get damaged, they die, and new cells take their place. Sometimes, this process goes wrong. New cells form when the body does not need them, and old or damaged cells fail to die as they should. The buildup of extra cells often forms a mass of tissue, which is referred to as a tumor.

Lung cancer cells can spread by breaking away from a lung tumor. These cells can travel through blood vessels or nodes to reach other parts of the body. This process is called metastasis. After spreading, cancer cells may attach to other tissues and grow to form new tumors that may damage their new host tissues. Not all cancer is the same, and some types are easier to control than others.

When lung cancer spreads from its original place to another part of the body, the new tumor has the same kind of abnormal cells and is referred to by the same name as the original, or primary, tumor. For example, if lung cancer spreads to the bones, the cancer cells in the bones are lung cancer cells. Therefore, this type of cancer, even though it is in the bone, is metastatic lung cancer, not bone cancer. In this situation, cancer that appears in the bone is treated as lung cancer, not bone cancer.

Types of Lung Cancer

Just as there are distinct types of cancer throughout the body, there are also distinct types of lung cancer. As a caregiver, it is essential that you know which type of lung cancer the person with cancer has been diagnosed with; treatment and all aspects of care depend on the type of lung cancer.

Small cell: The cells of small cell lung cancer look small under a microscope. About 1 out of every eight people with lung cancer has small cell lung cancer.

Non-small cell: The cells of non-small cell lung cancer are larger than the cells of small cell lung cancer. Most people, about 7 out of every 8 with lung cancer, have the non-small cell variety. Non-small cell lung cancer does not grow and spread as fast as small cell lung cancer, and the two types of lung cancer call for different treatments. Within non-small cell lung cancer, there are also two distinct classifications: adenocarcinoma and squamous cell cancer.

Staging of Lung Cancer

Staging is the assessment of the extent of spread of the tumor, including spread to lymph nodes and metastasis, when cancer spreads to other parts of the body. The oncologist who is treating the person with cancer will determine how to treat the cancer based on the stage and location in the body.

Staging tests that the person with cancer may undergo:

A biopsy: a small piece of tissue is taken from the patient's affected tissues and examined under a microscope.

CT scan: an x-ray machine linked to a computer takes a series of detailed pictures of the patient's chest, abdomen, brain, or other parts of the body. First, the patient receives an injection of contrast material in a blood vessel in the arm or hand. In some cases, the patient will also drink a solution containing contrast material. The contrast material makes abnormal areas easier to see on the scan. The pictures from a CT scan can help to determine the lung tumor's size. The scans can also help to show if cancer has spread to the liver, adrenal glands, brain, or other organs.

PET scan: the health care team of the person with cancer may order a PET scan to get a better view of the tumor in the lung or to find cancer that has spread to other parts of the body. The patient will receive an injection of a small amount of radioactive sugar before the scan. Then, a specialized machine creates computerized pictures of the sugar being used by cells in the body. Because cancer cells use sugar faster than normal cells, areas with cancer cells appear brighter.

MRI: a strong magnet linked to a computer is used to make detailed pictures of the patient's head or spine. An MRI can show whether cancer has spread to these areas. Sometimes contrast material is used to make abnormal areas show up more clearly on the image.

Bone scan: A small amount of a radioactive substance is injected into a blood vessel. The radioactive substance travels through the patient's bloodstream and collects in the bones. A machine called a scanner detects and measures the radiation. The scanner uses this data to create images of the patient's bones. Because higher amounts of the radioactive substance collect in areas where cancer is present, the images can help determine whether cancer has spread to the bones.

Stages for Non-Small Cell Lung Cancer

All non-small cell lung cancers are staged the same way, whether the tumor is determined to be adenocarcinoma or squamous cell lung cancer. See *Lung Cancer Choices, 5th Edition*, Chapter 1: Diagnosis and Staging of Lung Cancer

Stage 0

This is called in situ disease, meaning the cancer is "in place" and has not grown into nearby tissues and spread outside the lung.

Stage I

A small tumor that has not spread to any lymph nodes, making it possible for a surgeon to completely remove it. Stage I is divided into 2 substages based on the size of the tumor:

- Stage IA tumors are 3 centimeters (cm) or less in size.
- Stage IB tumors are more than 3 cm but 4 cm or less in size.

Stage II

Stage II lung cancer is divided into 2 substages:

- A stage IIA cancer describes a tumor larger than 4 cm but 5 cm or less in size that has not spread to the nearby lymph nodes.
- Stage IIB lung cancer describes a tumor that is 5 cm or less in size that has spread to the lymph nodes. A stage IIB cancer can also be a tumor more than 5 cm wide that has not spread to the lymph nodes.

Stage III

Stage III lung cancers are classified as either stage IIIA, IIIB, or IIIC. The stage is based on the size of the tumor and which lymph nodes the cancer has spread to. Stage III cancers have not spread to other distant parts of the body.

Stage IV

Stage IV means the lung cancer has spread to more than 1 area in the other lung, the fluid surrounding the lung or the heart, or distant parts of the body through the bloodstream.

Stages for Small Cell Lung Cancer

Most doctors describe the stages of small cell lung cancer with two stages:

Limited stage: Cancer is found only on one side of the chest.

Extensive stage: Cancer is found in the lung and also in tissues on the other side of the chest.

-OR-

Lung cancer is in distant organs, such as the brain, or the fluid between the two layers of pleura.

Additional Testing for Non-Small Cell Lung Cancer

Comprehensive Biomarker Testing

Lung cancer is a complex cancer that has known mutations. Biomarkers are molecules in the blood or tissue that can result from mutations in genes.

Biomarkers help to link subsets of people diagnosed with non-small cell lung cancer (NSCLC) to certain therapies and can help predict response, resistance, or toxicity to certain drugs. With improved biomarker testing techniques, an expanding list of molecular targets and more approved and emerging therapies, comprehensive biomarker testing is an essential part of the evaluation and management of all patients diagnosed with NSCLC. See *Lung Cancer Choices, 5th Edition*, Chapter 2: Comprehensive Biomarker Testing

Caregiver
CHOICES

CHAPTER 7

TREATMENTS FOR LUNG CANCER

Surgery

If the diagnosis is early-stage lung cancer, surgery may be an option. The surgeon usually removes only the part of the lung that contains cancer. Most people who have surgery for lung cancer will have the lobe of the lung that contains cancer removed. This procedure is called a lobectomy. In some cases, the surgeon will remove the tumor along with less tissue than an entire lobe or the surgeon will remove the entire lung. The surgeon also may remove nearby lymph nodes. See *Lung Cancer Choices, 5th Edition*, Chapter 1: Diagnosis and Staging of Lung Cancer

Radiation

Radiation therapy is an option for people with any stage of lung cancer:

- People with early lung cancer may choose radiation therapy instead of surgery.
- After surgery, radiation therapy can be used to try to destroy any cancer cells that may remain in the chest.
- In advanced lung cancer, they may use a combination of radiation therapy and chemotherapy. Radiation therapy can be used to help shrink a tumor that is blocking a patient's airway.

- Radiation therapy can be used to help relieve pain from lung cancer that has spread to the bones or other tissues.
- Radiation therapy is often used to treat lung cancer that has spread to the brain.

A large machine produces radiation during radiation therapy, which aims high-energy rays at the patient's body to kill cancer cells. The treatment affects cells only in the treatment area, such as the chest area.

The person with cancer will visit a hospital or clinic for radiation treatment. Radiation therapy usually consists of treatment five days per week for about six weeks. Each treatment session usually lasts less than 20 minutes.

Although radiation therapy is painless, it may cause significant side effects. The side effects depend mainly on the amount of radiation used and the location of the tumor. Encourage the person with cancer to ask his or her health care team to describe the side effects that might occur during or after radiation therapy. See *Lung Cancer Choices, 5th Edition*, Chapter 5: Radiation Therapy for Non-Small Cell Lung Cancer

Chemotherapy

Chemotherapy uses drugs to kill cancer cells. The drugs for lung cancer are usually administered intravenously, which means that they are injected directly into a vein using a thin needle.

The person with cancer will probably receive chemotherapy in a clinic or at a physician's office. Often there are reclining chairs for patients, and they rarely need to stay in the hospital during treatment.

The side effects of chemotherapy depend mainly on which drugs are administered and the dosage levels. Chemotherapy kills fast-growing cancer cells, but the drugs can also harm healthy cells that divide rapidly:

- Blood cells: When drugs lower the levels of healthy blood cells, the person with cancer is more likely to get infections, bruise or bleed easily, and feel very weak and tired. The patient's health care team will regularly check for low levels of blood cells. If the patient's levels are low, his or her health care team may stop the chemotherapy for some time or reduce the dose of the drug. They may also choose to prescribe medications that can help the patient's body create new blood cells.

- Cells in hair roots: Chemotherapy may cause hair loss. If the person with cancer loses his or her hair, it will grow back after treatment, but the color and texture may be changed.
- Cells that line the digestive tract: Chemotherapy can result in poor appetite, nausea and vomiting, diarrhea, or mouth and lip sores. The patient's health care team can prescribe medications and suggest other ways to help with these problems.

Targeted Therapies

Targeted cancer therapies block the growth and spread of cancer by interfering with specific molecules involved in tumor growth and progression. By focusing on molecular and cellular changes that are specific to cancer, targeted cancer therapies may be more effective than other types of treatment, but there are not targeted therapies for all types of cancer and at all stages. See *Lung Cancer Choices, 5th Edition*, Chapter 4: Systemic Therapy for Non-Small Cell Lung Cancer (Chemotherapy, Targeted Therapy, and Immunotherapy)

Smoking Cessation

If you smoke, many studies have shown improved survival from lung cancer in patients who stop smoking compared to those who do not. The person with cancer may want to continue smoking; being diagnosed with a serious disease is stressful. Smoking is addictive, due to the nicotine in tobacco, and it is hard for most smokers to quit in the best of times. Many patients fall back on smoking as a coping mechanism that is familiar to them. Encourage the person with cancer to ask about smoking cessation resources from his or her health care team. See *Lung Cancer Choices, 5th Edition,* Chapter 13: How to Quit Smoking Confidently and Successfully

To find out more about the specific medicines that the person with cancer is receiving, we again recommend the reliable and thorough resources on the National Cancer Institute's website: https://www.cancer.gov/about-cancer/treatment/drugs/lung

Caregiver
CHOICES

CHAPTER 8

LUNG CANCER HEALTH CARE TEAM

The Multi-Disciplinary Lung Cancer Team

Lung cancer can cause a great deal of uncertainty, but there is a team of highly trained professionals whose job it is to help the person with cancer through these difficult times. The number of people whom a person with lung cancer will meet and the information that he or she will receive about therapy can be overwhelming and confusing. As a caregiver, you should try to meet as many of the members of the health care team as possible so that you can fully support the person with cancer along his or her journey.

As you are developing your team you may hear the term integrative oncology. Integrative oncology is a patient-centered, evidence-informed field of cancer care that utilizes mind and body practices, natural products, and/or lifestyle modifications from different traditions alongside conventional cancer treatments. Integrative oncology aims to optimize health, quality of life, and clinical outcomes across the cancer care continuum and to empower people to prevent cancer and become active participants before, during, and beyond cancer treatment

The following information provides a brief overview of members of the cancer care team.

Pulmonologist

A pulmonologist, or lung doctor, is a physician who specializes in diseases of the airway and lungs. If the person with cancer is found to have one or more nodules, sometimes referred to as 'spots', on his or her lungs based on a chest x-ray or a CT scan, then a pulmonologist may be one of the first physicians the patient will see. A pulmonologist's focus is to aid in reaching a diagnosis, including helping to determine whether the nodule seems to be lung cancer. The patient's consultation with a pulmonologist may include various procedures, such as bronchoscopy and biopsies.

Radiologist

A radiologist is a physician who specializes in reading body imaging including, x-rays, computed tomography (CT) scans, and Positron Emission Tomography (PET) scans. Radiologists help diagnose lung cancer and can perform CT-guided biopsies of tumors. A radiologist and a radiation oncologist are different doctors with distinct specialties.

Radiation Oncologist

Radiation oncologists are physicians who specialize in the use of radiation therapy to treat cancer. The focus of radiation oncologists is to help design a treatment plan and direct radiation therapy. Radiation oncologists work closely with an array of other health care providers, including radiation oncology nurses, medical physicists, radiation therapists, and dosimetrists. Radiation oncologists will help the person with cancer choose the most effective radiation therapy for his or her specific cancer.

Medical Oncologist

Medical oncologists are physicians who specialize in systemic therapy, including chemotherapy, targeted therapy, and immunotherapy, for the treatment of cancer. The person with cancer may meet a medical oncologist in an outpatient clinic or the hospital. A Medical oncologist will determine if the person with cancer is a candidate for therapy, what type of therapy he or she will receive, and the duration of treatment. Medical oncologists will frequently monitor the condition of the person with cancer while he or she is receiving treatment and will help minimize the side effects of treatment.

Thoracic Surgeons

Thoracic surgeons are physicians who specialize in chest surgery, which includes the chest wall, mediastinum, lungs, esophagus, and diaphragm. Thoracic surgeons perform diagnostic procedures and surgical treatment for patients with lung cancer. During the patient's evaluation, the surgeons will assess how fit the person with cancer is for surgery. This determination may involve obtaining laboratory tests or specialized studies. Before treatment, thoracic surgeons will discuss the options for surgery and will be the primary physician managing the patient's care in the hospital after surgery.

Palliative Care Team

> *We should have had palliative care from the beginning.*
> *-Jan*

Palliative medicine is a relatively new medical specialty that can assist with symptom management, including general pain, nerve pain, shortness of breath, and fatigue. Palliative care physicians can help families, and caregivers navigate the complex medical environment. A palliative care physician can be especially helpful by offering valuable assistance with decisions at crucial points in treatment. Palliative care can be provided at any time in the course of the cancer care, including during active treatment.

Physician Assistant or Nurse Practitioner

Physician assistants (PA) and nurse practitioners (NP) are medical professionals who work as part of the care team both in both the outpatient clinic and in the hospital. When the plan is straightforward during treatment, the person with cancer may regularly see a PA or an NP instead of his or her oncologist.

Oncology Nurse

Every oncologist has a specially trained nurse who works with the person with cancer to provide practical coping skills for dealing with the effects of cancer and the treatments. The oncology nurse can be a valuable partner for caregivers.

Oncology Registered Dietitian

An oncology registered dietitian helps to address nutrition issues that become barriers to healing in treatment.

Social Worker

A social worker has the training to help patients deal with mental, emotional, and daily living issues. Social workers take care of the connections with other agencies, including home health providers, infusion companies, oxygen and medical equipment agencies, and hospice providers. Social workers can also help the person with cancer determine whether he or she is eligible for government programs or other aid. Social workers are trained to counsel patients about grief and coping issues. A social worker can also assist you and the person with cancer, manage important legal matters, such as developing Durable Power of Attorney and Living Will documents.

Kinesiologist or Physical Therapist

A kinesiologist is a regulated health professional that treats and prevents injury, disease and improves health and wellness. Kinesiologists address the physiological and mechanical systems of the body. The main objective for a kinesiologist is to help you live a more functional and pain free life. It's best to choose a kinesiologist if you have a condition, injury or disability you need help dealing with as they can help you improve your fitness and mobility.

A physical therapist is a health professional that helps with treatment or management of physical disability, malfunction, or pain by exercise, massage, hydrotherapy, etc., without the use of medicines, surgery, or radiation.

For a lung cancer patient, putting together his or her health care team will involve a lot of difficult choices. As a caregiver, you can help the patient make these decisions in an organized and logical manner. Encourage the person with cancer to include all factors directly or indirectly involved in care. For example, the person with cancer might be struggling with a decision to see a highly regarded medical oncologist at a university hospital in the next state or staying with the local, community oncologist.

You can help the person with cancer make this choice by helping him or her construct a simple list of the advantages for each option, making sure that you include practical issues that will affect daily life: Should we go to a university oncologist or an oncologist in our community?

Advantages of university oncologist	*Advantages of oncologist closer to home*
Specializes in a type of cancer	Treatments are standardized so that would be the same
Access to clinical trials	Closer communication with your physician
Access to specialized surgeons, radiation oncologists	Less burden on travel (time, costs) for patient and family

It is especially important to inform each of your health care providers about all the treatment approaches you are using. This is particularly important if you choose an integrative medicine approach that involves health care providers or treatments from several different medical providers.

Clinical Trials

At their heart, clinical trials are research to benefit future lung cancer patients. The person with cancer may choose to explore clinical trial options as a generous gesture, hoping that he or she can contribute to advancing the science of lung cancer care. Sometimes it is possible that a clinical trial can offer immediate help to patients participating in the trial by providing access to potential new treatments. Clinical trials are usually offered when current therapies are sub-optimal or when no proven therapies are available. If the person with cancer decides to participate in a clinical trial, he or she will, at the very least, be watched closely and receive treatment from clinicians dedicated to advancing lung cancer treatments. Even if the health of the person with cancer does not directly improve being in the clinical trial, he or she may find peace of mind and pride knowing that the trial will help develop treatments for future patients. See *Lung Cancer Choices, 5th Edition*, Chapter 7: Clinical Trials and Emerging Therapies for Lung Cancer

Clinical trials, including those used to develop cancer treatments, are the final step in a long process to test new drugs or other therapies. Testing of a new cancer drug or treatment is an orderly series of steps called phases. This process allows researchers to obtain reliable information about the drug or treatment to protect patients in each part of the study.

Understanding the different phases of clinical trials can help you provide sound advice to the person with cancer if he or she is considering joining a study.

- **Phase 1 trials:** Researchers test a new drug or treatment in a small group of people for the first time to evaluate its safety, determine a safe dosage range, and identify side effects.
- **Phase 2 trials:** The focus of phase 2 trials is safety. During this phase, researchers determine whether the drug or treatment is effective in people who have a specific disease or condition. For example, participants receiving the new drug or treatment may be compared with similar participants receiving the current standard of care or a different drug or treatment.
- **Phase 3 trials:** In a phase 3 clinical trial, the drug or treatment is administered to a large group of people to confirm effectiveness, monitor side effects, compare to commonly used drugs or treatments, and collect information that will allow the drug or treatment to be utilized safely.

- **Phase 4 trials:** Phase 4 studies are conducted after a drug or treatment has been approved for use in the general public. Phase 4 trials are conducted to provide more information about side effects, long-term risks and benefits, and effectiveness in the general population.

Notes

Caregiver
CHOICES

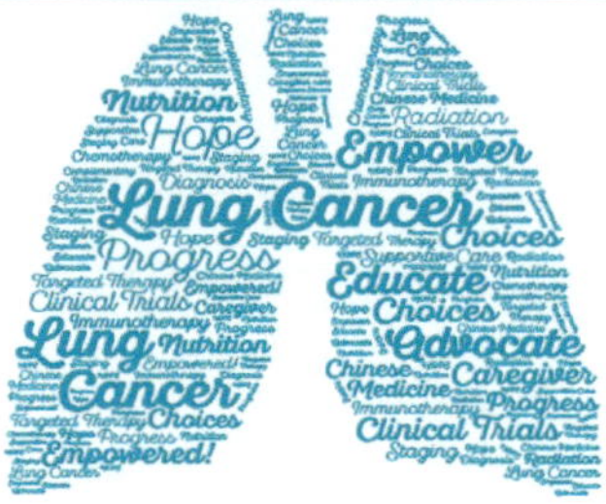

CHAPTER 9

QUESTIONS FOR THE HEALTH CARE TEAM

At various points throughout the process, the person with cancer will have many questions for his or her health care team. Almost all health care professionals are competent and caring and have their patients' best interest at heart, but they cannot anticipate the needs of every single one of their patients throughout their busy days. As a caregiver, you can help the person with cancer prepare for visits with members of their health care team by developing a list of questions beforehand, rather than hoping that the right questions will come to mind once he or she is in the room with the provider. There are many different questions that may become important at different times—help the person with cancer write down a list to bring along to each appointment. These do not need to be complicated or fancy questions.

Here are some sample questions to help you and the person with cancer get started:

- Where is my tumor located? Can you show me on the image?
- What stage is my cancer?
- Can my cancer be cured?

- What is the treatment plan?
- What is the schedule of the therapy?
- How long are the various treatments?
- What are the potential side effects?
- How will these side effects be managed?
- Can you provide paperwork for the caregiver's workplace so that the caregiver can come to the appointments?
- Are the treatments covered by insurance and who can help me check?
- What integrative, alternative, or complementary therapies are worth exploring?
- Who is the primary contact at the clinic if my family needs to talk to someone?
- Is this illness related to my military service?
- Who is the after-hours contact?
- Should we look into consulting a specialist in lung cancer?
- Should we go to a university oncologist or an oncologist in our community?
- What expectations are there for the caregiver?

It can be hard to remember all of the questions that you may have for your health care team. Caring Ambassadors offers Lung Cancer Question Builder. It is a tool designed to take you through a series of questions you may want to ask your health care team as you navigate the journey ahead. You can print out your questions and take it with you, or email it to your provider ahead of time. Being prepared will help you better communicate with your health care team.

Caregiver
CHOICES

CHAPTER 10

PROGNOSIS

Sometimes patients and families ask, "How long am I (or my loved one) going to live?" Of course, it is unlikely that the health care team will be able to answer this question with any level of accuracy—every patient is different, and so is the course of the disease. However, some averages can provide general guidance. Even if the person with cancer is given an estimate, the actual outcome will depend heavily on several issues including, but not limited to:

- Response to treatment
- How well the patient is getting up and around
- The human spirit and attitude

> *Every patient is different and so is the course of the disease.*

For some patients, it is personally important for them to have a prognosis. Some people want to plan ahead as much as possible, get their financial affairs in order, and change their priorities depending on the expected outcome of the disease and the associated timeline. For others, a prognosis only causes fear and anxiety for both the patient his or her loved ones. As a caregiver, you should follow the lead of the person with cancer; make sure that the patient gets all of the information that he or she wants, but do not push a prognosis on someone who is not ready. For some people with lung cancer, understanding a broad range of potential outcomes and timelines is more helpful. Regardless, you can encourage the person with cancer to live every day fully while also starting to put his or her affairs in order.

Caregiver
CHOICES

CHAPTER 11

KEY DECISION POINTS IN CARE

At any time, the person with cancer can ask the members of his or her health care team to sit down and explain the big picture or where things stand. One practical approach is to encourage the person with cancer to explain to the health care team his or her understanding of the current situation and the road ahead. This approach allows the patient to get a fuller picture of the situation by using his or her own words to describe where things stand. The members of the health care team can then correct any misunderstandings to make sure that the person with cancer and every member of his or her health care team are all on the same page.

> ***Lung cancer can cause a great deal of uncertainty. Do not hesitate to ask questions at any time in the process.***

Again, the person with cancer can request a "big picture" conversation at any time. However, there are certain decision points at which you, as a caregiver, may want to encourage such discussions:

- At diagnosis
- Before treatment begins
- After completion of radiation therapy

- After completion of chemotherapy
- Any time that the treatment has not been successful

Caregiver
CHOICES

CONCLUSION

When someone you care for has a lung cancer diagnosis, it can have a significant impact on your life. You will be bombarded with advice and information about caring for someone with cancer, and it is easy to get lost in all of the changes to your world. While we hope that you might find many helpful hints in this book, if you only take one thing away from reading it, we hope that it is this: take care of yourself.

It is natural for a caregiver to want to concentrate only on the person with cancer, but this is not healthy for anyone involved. It is not selfish to look out for yourself: taking care of your own needs will make you a more effective caregiver. As a caregiver, you may experience periods of stress, frustration, and even depression. Do not ignore these feelings in yourself. Learn to recognize signs that you are not feeling 100 percent and then act. You can find support from others who are caregivers or talk to a professional. You can ask others to share the load, either by helping care for the person with cancer directly or by taking over some of your daily tasks. You can make time for yourself by scheduling fun activities away from the person with cancer.

In addition to being emotionally taxing, being a caregiver can take a real physical toll as well. Make sure that you take time to take care of your body. Do not get so caught up in your caregiving responsibilities that you neglect your physical health. Take time away to exercise, to eat decent meals, and to get enough sleep.

Finally, as a caregiver, do not be too hard on yourself. Make sure that you confer all of the good, positive emotions that you feel for the person with cancer to yourself as well. Be kind, forgiving, and patient with yourself. Being a caregiver for a person with lung cancer is a challenging role to play and you can only do so much. Cut yourself a little slack and make sure that you look out for your well-being. Taking care of yourself is not in any way neglecting the person with cancer; anything that you can do to maintain your health will be better for both you and the person with cancer.

Caregiver
CHOICES

CAREGIVER RESOURCES (ONLINE)

Caring Ambassadors Program

The Caring Ambassadors Program is a non-profit organization with a singular mission: to improve the lives of patients and communities by empowering and educating them to be advocates for their own health.

503 632 9032

https://caringambassadors.org

Caregiver Action Network

The Caregiver Action Network serves a broad spectrum of family caregivers ranging from the parents of children with special needs, to the families and friends of wounded soldiers; from a young couple dealing with a diagnosis of MS, to adult children caring for parents with Alzheimer's disease.

800 896 3650

www.caregiveraction.org

Eldercare Locator

Are you a family caregiver in need of information or assistance? Are you interested in learning more about the programs and services that may be of assistance to you or your loved one? The Eldercare Locator, a public service of the U.S. Administration on Aging, is the first step to finding resources for older adults in any U.S. community. Just one phone call or Website visit provides an instant connection to resources that enable older persons to live independently in their communities. The service links those who need assistance with state and local area agencies on aging and community-based

organizations that serve older adults and their caregivers.
www.eldercare.acl.gov

Family Reach
Family Reach is a financial lifeline for families fighting cancer.
www.FamilyReach.org

Financial Steps for Caregivers
WISER (Women's Institute for a Secure Retirement)

Financial Steps for Caregivers: What You Need to Know About Money and Retirement is designed to help you identify financial decisions you may face as a caregiver. The decision to become a caregiver can affect both your short-term and long-term financial security, including your own retirement.
www.wiserwomen.org

Foundation for Financial Planning
To help people take control of their financial lives by connecting the financial planning community to people in need.
www.Foundationforfinancialplanning.org

Family Caregiver Alliance
Family Caregiver Alliance supports and sustains the important work of families nationwide caring for loved ones with chronic, disabling health conditions.
800 445 8106
www.caregiver.org

My Choices: A Planner for Healing
My Choices will help empower you to create, track and research your own journey to wellness.
https://caringambassadors.org

National Alliance for Caregiving
Established in 1996, The National Alliance for Caregiving is a non-profit coalition of national organizations focusing on issues of family caregiving.
www.caregiving.org

Next Step in Care

Next Step in Care provides easy-to-use guides to help family caregivers and health care providers work closely together to plan and implement safe and smooth transitions for chronically or seriously ill patients.

www.nextstepincare.org

Well Spouse Association

Providing peer support and education about the special challenges and unique issues facing "well" spouses every day.

www.wellspouse.org

Notes

Caregiver
CHOICES

AFTERWORD

A Message from Caring Ambassadors Lung Cancer Program Director, Cindy Langhorne-Hatfield.

There are always "choices and hope" for all people facing lung cancer, whether you are living with the disease yourself or are the loved one of someone who is. For many people, hope grows when you have the information and support you need to make health care decisions that suit your personal goals and circumstances. At Caring Ambassadors, we are dedicated to helping improve the overall wellness of people living with lung cancer through information, education, and personal choice.

The good news is that lung cancer treatment and management options have changed dramatically over the past decade through the addition of new targeted therapies and immunotherapy drug options. Testing to detect specific biomarkers has become more common as precision medicine continues to evolve. With more treatment options approved for various types and stages of lung cancer, it is important to understand all your treatment options.

Caring Ambassadors is honored to be serving the lung cancer community. Please do not hesitate to reach out for more information at: info@lungcancercap.org

Don't miss Caring Ambassadors Program's

Lung Cancer Choices, 5th Edition

Lung Cancer Choices is written with several purposes in mind:

- to provide information about lung cancer to help you make decisions about lung cancer treatment options.
- to provide a balanced view of the currently available treatment options from Western medicine, complementary and alternative medicine (CAM), and Chinese medicine.
- to help you communicate more effectively with healthcare providers.
- to help you become empowered to be the best advocate for your healthcare.

Making Informed Decisions Potentially life-changing decisions are one aspect of having a serious illness such as lung cancer. Each of us is unique in how we make decisions. Some people want to know everything they possibly can about their disease and make all their own treatment decisions. Other people prefer to have their healthcare providers make treatment decisions based on their knowledge and expertise. Some prefer having a friend or family member seek out and sort through information. Many use a combination of approaches.

We hope Lung Cancer Choices will help you understand your disease and some of the health care options available to you. Knowledge empowers you to ask the necessary questions to become your own best advocate. When your questions have been asked and answered, you and your healthcare providers will be in the best possible situation to determine the best treatment approach for you.

Caregiver
CHOICES

ABOUT THE CONTRIBUTING AUTHORS

Dr. Ann Broderick graduated with an AB in Latin American literature from Princeton University. She is a 1986 graduate of the Carver College of Medicine and completed residency in Internal Medicine in 1989 at the University of Iowa Hospitals and Clinics. She then worked as a general internist and a hospice medical director. After 10 years in that position, she became the Director of Palliative care at University of Iowa Hospital and Clinics. She is currently the Director of Hospice and Palliative Care at the VA Medical Center in Iowa City.

Dr. Broderick has been a tireless champion of patient and family education, as she feels that patients can collaborate best with their health care teams when they are informed. Lung cancer patients and their families have contributed greatly to her understanding of the full impact of this disease. She continues to work with oncologists to control symptoms during cancer treatment in her role as a palliative care physician at the VA Medical Center.

Fred LaBrecque worked as the Medical Writer and Program Development Director for the Caring Ambassadors. He has experience in all facets of the medical research field: basic laboratory research, clinical trials, data coordination, and program management. In his work, Fred has written and edited a variety of publications, from editorials aimed at general audiences, to scholarly articles published in peer-reviewed journals.

Notes

Caregiver
CHOICES

ABOUT THE EDITORS

Fred LaBrecque worked as the Medical Writer and Program Development Director for the Caring Ambassadors. He has experience in all facets of the medical research field: basic laboratory research, clinical trials, data coordination, and program management. In his work, Fred has written and edited a variety of publications, from editorials aimed at general audiences, to scholarly articles published in peer-reviewed journals.

Cindy Langhorne-Hatfield joined the Caring Ambassadors Program, Inc. in August of 2007 as the Lung Cancer Program Director. Ms. Langhorne-Hatfield brings over twenty-four years of programmatic and managerial experience in the field of lung cancer advocacy and has worked with public and private community stakeholders. Ms. Langhorne-Hatfield's compassion for lung cancer patients and their families and her dedication to improving the burdens of lung cancer one life at a time are extraordinary. Ms. Langhorne-Hatfield is a well-respected local, regional, and national advocate for lung cancer and issues that affect those living with or at risk for the disease.

Ms. Langhorne-Hatfield is also the acting Co-Chair for the Lung Cancer Action Network (LungCAN®). The Lung Cancer Action Network (LungCAN®) is a collaborative group of lung cancer advocacy organizations and patient driven biomarker groups who have come together to raise public awareness of the realities of lung cancer to increase funding for detecting, treating and curing the disease.

Notes

Caregiver
CHOICES

ACKNOWLEDGMENTS

The Caring Ambassadors Lung Cancer Program is profoundly grateful to the author Ann Broderick, MD, MS, Director, Hospice and Palliative Care for her expertise in making this a reality. Without Dr. Broderick's commitment to this project, we would be unable to offer this important resource to the lung cancer community. We would also like to thank Fred LaBrecque, Caring Ambassadors former Medical Writer and Program Development Director for his expertise in medial editing and writing.

Like a family, the Caring Ambassadors Lung Cancer Program has a core of support upon which it stands and draws on for strength. Caregiver Choices would not be possible without the love and generosity of our dedicated Board members and their families. Thank you for all you do for the Caring Ambassadors Program and the community.

Last but not least, the Caring Ambassadors Lung Cancer Program acknowledges the lung cancer community —the people who bravely face the challenges of living with lung cancer. The loved ones who offer them steadfast support and comfort. The health care providers who work to provide the best possible treatment options. The advocates who work tirelessly to provide hope, support, and improve the future for those at risk for developing lung cancer and those living with the disease. We are proud to work side-by-side with you to meet the community's needs.

Thank you to our sponsors for their generous support of our educational materials.

Made in United States
Cleveland, OH
19 October 2026

46341972R00043